EAT THE RIGHT FOODS
FOR OPTIMUM HEALTH :

These nutritional foods are reasonably priced for any budget.

"Let food be thy medicine and medicine be thy food" ~Hippocrates

BY   S.ELIA

The greatest wealth is Health." ~Unknown

1. Eating smart will not only make you smart, it's the smart thing to do.

Eating right does wonders for your body.

"If you don't take care of your body, where are you
going to live?" ~Unknown

"Take care of your body. It's the only place you
have to live."
~Jim Rohn

Disclaimer: This book is for information   how
to eat the right foods for optimum health. However
if you have any allergies or sensitivities to any of
the foods I mention , avoid eating those foods that
do not agree with your body. If you get any

reaction to any food whether I mention it in this
book or not, you should consult your trusted doctor
for proper advice, diagnosis and treatment .

The author
S.ELIA

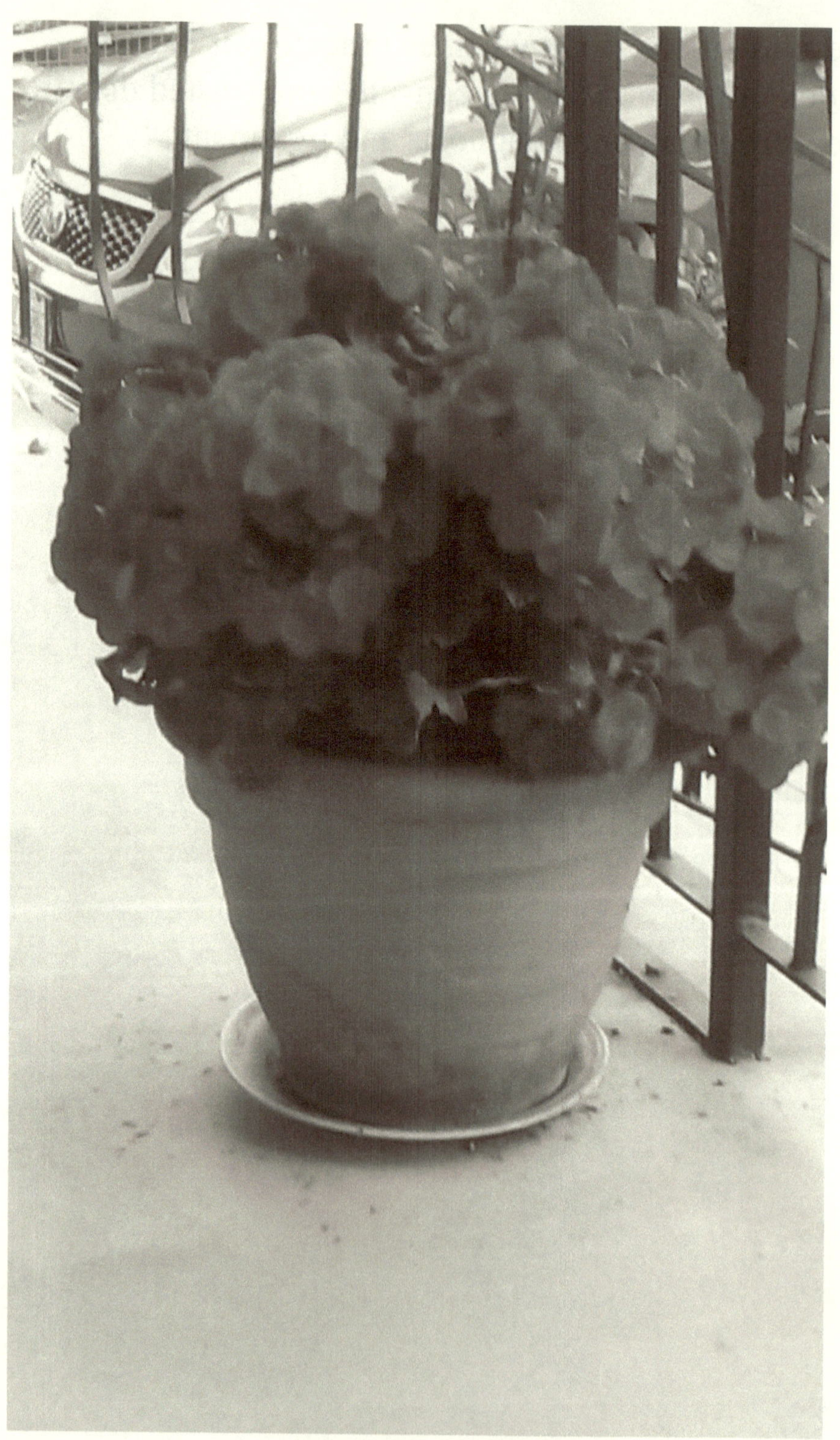

PROLOGUE.

Every day millions of people   spend huge amounts
of money to eat refined junk foods starving their
bodies from the proper nutrients ending up
overfed, fat and undernourished. Others spend a
lot of money   feeding their addictions, smoking,
drinking , doing drugs or other addictions and
neglect their nutritional needs.
The responsibility and the number one job of
every living creature is to keep their bodies in good
health by eating nutritional foods. Unfortunately
most people either do not know enough about
nutrition or they just ignore their bodies nutritional
needs.
In this book, I will try to explain to anyone who
is willing to listen that you do not have to spend a
lot of money to eat nutritional food. As a matter of
fact the most nutritional foods are relatively cheap
and anyone can eat GOOD FOOD at any budget!

THE BEST FOODS ARE REASONABLY PRICED

 Rich or frugal budgets can afford to buy and enjoy the best nutritional foods on the market. These foods provide all the nutritional needs of humans at any age.

THE BEST FOOD

The best food of all is, did you guessed it? IT IS THE MILK, the first food we have after we are born.

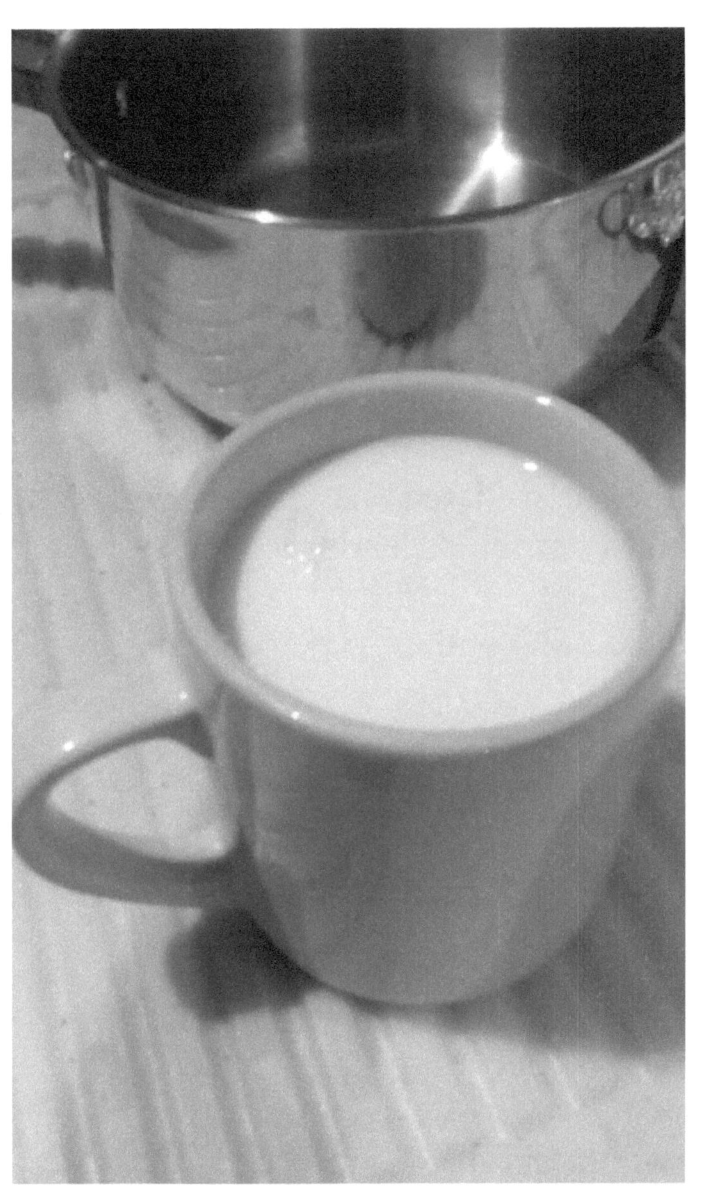

Milk has all the ingredients to sustain life. Babies live their first few months of life by drinking only milk from their mother's breasts, breastfeeding or milk from a bottle usually cows milk.
Milk INCLUDING cow's milk contains protein, which supports muscle growth and repair and many vitamins and minerals which are essential for the bodily functions.

Nutritional content of milk.

One cup of milk is considered one serving. The nutritional values of milk depends on the fat content.
One cup of whole milk, with 3.25 percent fat contains:

- 146 calories
- 8 grams of fat
- 13 grams of carbohydrates
- 8 grams of protein

One cup of skim milk contains:

- 86 calories
- 0 grams of fat
- 12 grams of carbohydrates
- 8 grams of protein

You can also have alternatives to cow's milk such as soy milk or almond milk for people that have *lactose intolerance.*

Lactose intolerance is a condition in which a person lacks the enzyme lactase, which is needed to break down the sugar found in milk for proper digestion.

A question arises for those people with lactose intolerance. How did they survived their early days of life when they were fed just milk for the first six months of their lives. Is it possible that they have lactose intolerance because they drink the milk cold and when they were babies, they were drinking warm milk, either warm milk from their mother or boiled cow's milk?

I think it is worth exploring this possibility. People with lactose intolerance should try drinking warm milk or boiled milk mixed with something else like oats or whole wheat toasts and see if they still have milk intolerance…..if they really have milk intolerance they should avoid milk or get some liquid lactase replacement. These are over-the-counter drops that you add to milk but you better ask your doctor for diagnosis and treatment.

one cup of plain soy milk contains:
- 80-110 calories
- 3 to 4 grams of fat

- 6 to 7 grams of carbohydrates
- 5 to 7 grams of protein

One cup of almond milk contains:

- 50 to 60 calories
- 2.5 grams of fat
- 5 to 7 grams of carbohydrates
- 1 gram of protein

Some important nutrients that all milk products provide include:

Calcium: Dairy products like milk are one of the richest dietary sources of calcium. Calcium has many functions in the body but the main function is for the maintenance of healthy bones. 99 percent of calcium is in the bones, and teeth but calcium plays key roles in blood clotting, muscle contraction and helps the heart, nerves and other body systems to work properly.

Daily calcium requirement is about 1000-1500mg and one cup of milk contains about 300mg.

Milk has nine essential nutrients including:

B vitamins (riboflavin, B-12 and niacin) for the conversion of food to energy.

High-quality protein is important for the maintenance and repair of muscles.

Vitamin A is important for healthy eyes and healthy immune system of the body.

Potassium is important in regulating the balance of fluids

Phosphorus, Calcium and Vitamin D   are essential for healthy strong   bones and other function of the body.

Drinking Milk everyday provides enough calcium for   the body's calcium needs. If not enough calcium is taken with the daily diet, it can lead to calcium deficiency and can cause mild or serious   symptoms.

A few symptoms of Calcium Deficiency. Calcium is the most abundant mineral in the body and it is essential   for the maintenance of strong bones and healthy teeth . Calcium deficiency occurs when there is not enough calcium intake   from the daily diet and can cause a variety of symptoms from mild to severe and life threatening including rickets and osteoporosis. Low blood calcium can lead to the following

low calcium symptoms.
Fainting, heart failure, chest pains, muscle cramps in the back and legs ,wheezing, seizures, dry skin, chronic itching, tooth decay, numbness and tingling in the extremities, osteoporosis with risk of fractures of the spine and other bones of the extremities.
That is the reason why people should have enough calcium in their daily diets and drinking milk every day   can prevent calcium deficiency. If there, is a problem with drinking milk try eating other foods rich in calcium such as
Cheese, Yogurt, Sardines, Dark leafy greens like spinach, kale, turnips?

Milk is best consumed warm   and never cold unless you live in a very hot climate, and even there you should boil the milk to avoid any food poisoning from bacteria contamination.. The human stomach tolerates better warm food that cold food. If milk causes a bloated stomach or gas in your abdomen consider drinking your milk warm with some honey or take it with other ingredients like whole wheat toast or oats or cereals.

Milk is good at any time of the day and you can have it as a drink or as prepared food with other ingredients.

 You should always boil raw milk to kill any

germs that might be present from any contamination.
Although pasteurized milk is supposed to be germ free it is still a good idea to boil it to kill any germs that might be present from any possible contamination from any source.
Besides warm milk is better than cold milk and it is tolerated better by the stomach.

@@@@@@@@@@@@@@@@@@@@@@@@
@@@@

Here are some suggestions how to consume milk daily with these simple recipes. You do not have to be a master chef to prepare these simple but very nutritious recipes.

FOR BREAKFAST

Milk and toast recipe
  for breakfast good for any age , young and old.
Ingredients
  1 CUP OF 2% MILK or 1% milk your choice

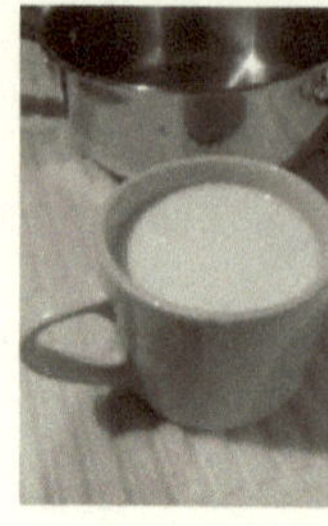

a cup of milk

2 SLICES OF WHOLE WHEAT BREAD toasted
or not.

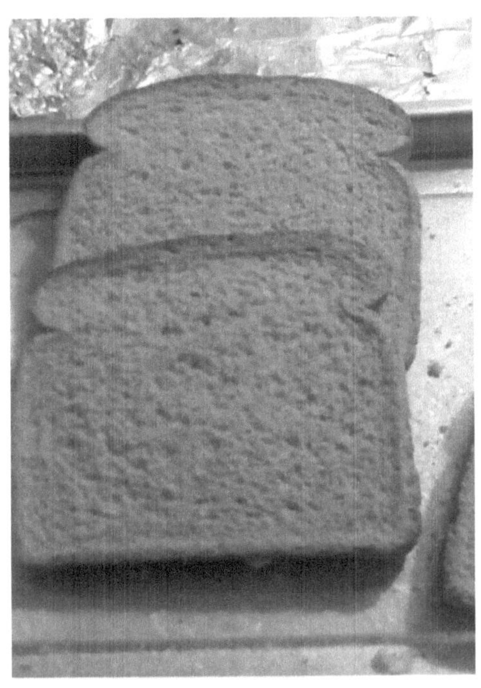

With the option of a tea spoon of honey or plain sugar for sweetening.

Pour the milk into a small pot and put it on the stove for 3-5 minutes until the milk warms up or boils. Be careful not to let it overflow the pot.

In a big cup put the two crumbled toasts and pour in the hot milk.

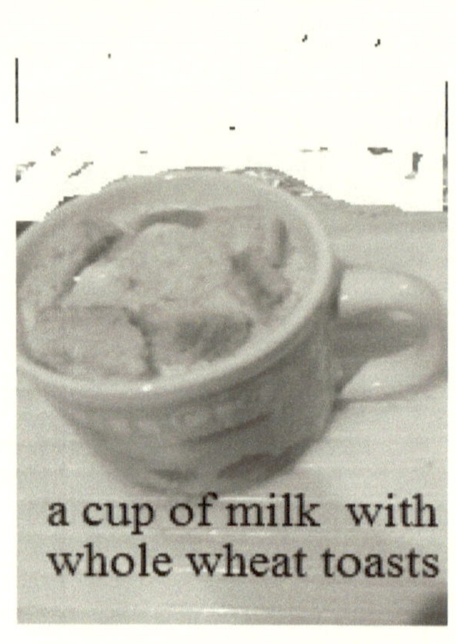

a cup of milk with
whole wheat toasts

Add a teaspoon of honey and stir well.
Stir and let it cool for a few minutes and then
using a table spoon eat the crumbled toasts with
the milk.
Should taste delicious. If you have a sweet tooth
you can add two tea spoons of honey in it.
This is a delicious and nutritious breakfast for
anybody OF ANY AGE but especially for the
young and old people.
Alternatively you can have just the warm milk
with the one tea spoon of honey which is a
delicious drink for breakfast.

SUGGESTION FOR CONSTIPATION
TREATMENT.

If you are suffering from constipation add 1-2
table spoons of bran into the milk or your bowl of
soup.
You can also add a table spoon of wheat germ. Stir
it well and eat it.
You can also take the bran and wheat germ into
a glass of orange juice and drink it.
By taking bran and wheat germ daily mixed in a
drink or with your food, will help you with
constipation but you have to take it daily. Besides
wheat, bran has dietary Fiber, Niacin, Vitamin B6,
Iron, Magnesium, Phosphorus, Zinc, Copper,
Manganese and Selenium.
Wheat germ is a great source of vegetable proteins,
along with fiber and healthy fats. It's also a good
source of magnesium, zinc, thiamin, folate,
potassium, and phosphorus. *Wheat germ* is high in
vitamin E, an essential *nutrient* with antioxidant
properties.
 By taking wheat bran and wheat germ will help
you with constipation and provides protein,
carbohydrates, vitamins and minerals which are
essential for the bodily functions.

SUGGESTION FOR HELP WITH INSOMNIA.

Drinking milk will help you sleep better.
If you are suffering from insomnia and

you have trouble sleeping at night try this simple solution.

Before going to your bed for your night sleep, boil a cup of milk 2% or 1% your choice let it cool for a few minutes, pour it into a cup add one teaspoon of liquid honey, stir it well and drink it. This simple recipe will help you sleep well at night. Milk will help you overcome your insomnia and your sleepless nights. Keep drinking milk every evening before you go to bed and you will be sleeping very well at night and you will be feeling very good as well. Milk has essential nutrients for good health.

@@@@@@@@@@@@@@@@@@@@@
@@@@

Another good meal for breakfast is milk   with oats.
 Milk and oats recipe ,
 good for any time of the day as a full meal.

Ingredients

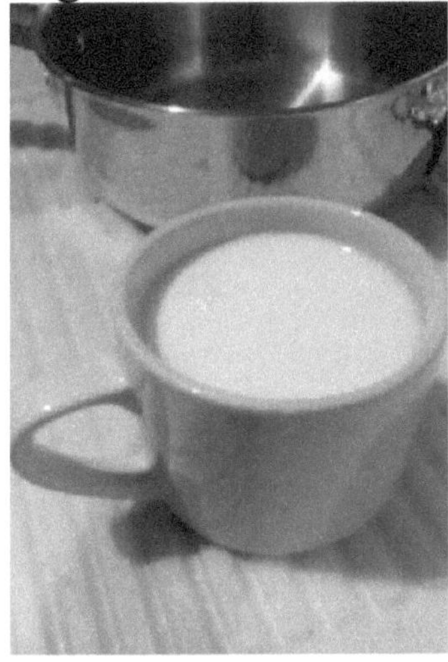

a cup of milk

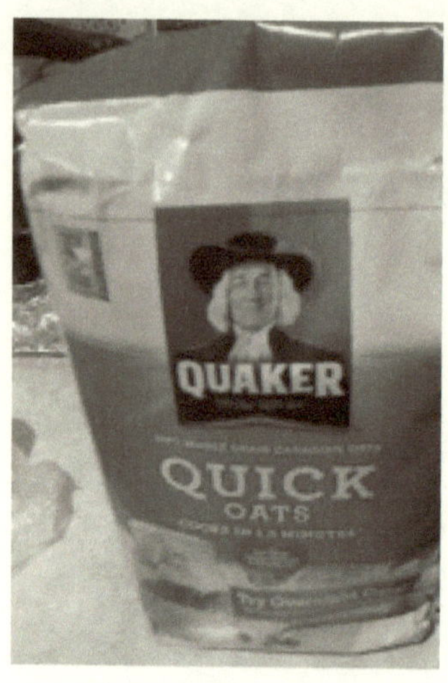

One cup of milk

One cup of water
one cup of quick or large flake oats
1 tea spoon of honey optional
1-2 table spoons of wheat bran and a tea spoon of
wheat germ if you are suffering from constipation
Pour the milk and the water in a pot and put it on
the stove.
When the mixture of milk and water starts to rise
just before it boils, add the one cup of instant oats.
Stir them well and keep stirring the mixture for
three to five minutes with a wooden spoon. Take
the pot off the stove and let it cool for three
minutes and serve it on a plate.

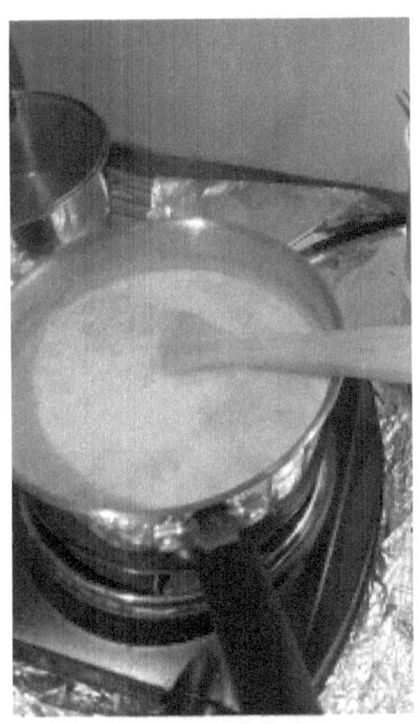

This is a delicious and nutritious fast meal for breakfast or any time of the day where you want a delicious food fast.

@@@@@@@@@@@@@@@@@@@@@@@@@@@@@@@

Recipe
Milk , oats and capellini pasta for a delicious meal.

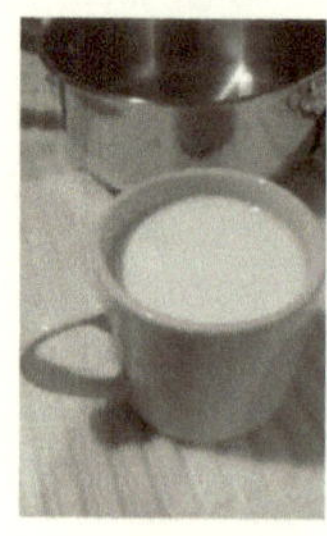
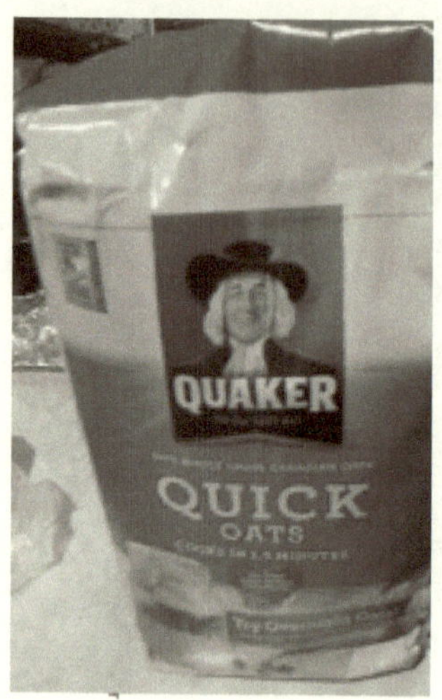

a cup of milk

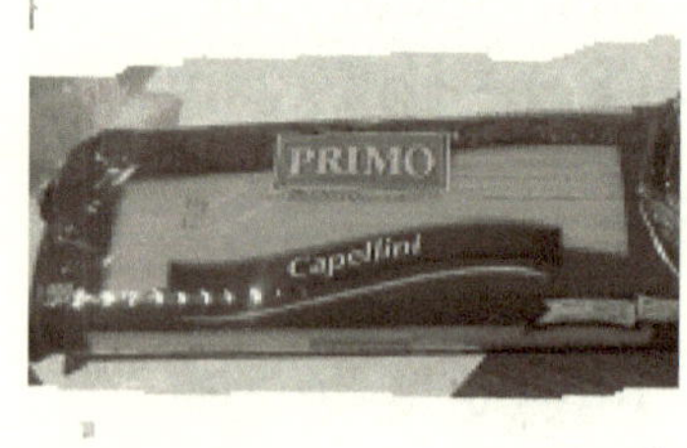

Ingredients , one cup of 2% milk and
 two cups of water
½ cup of oats
½ cup of capellini pasta broken into 1 inch
pieces
Optional one teaspoon of honey
Optional 1-2 table spoons of bran and one
teaspoon of wheat germ

Pour the milk and the water in a pot and place it on
the stove

When the mixture   rises and starts to boil
Add the oats and the pasta and keep stirring the
mixture for   5-6 minutes with a wooden spoon. If it
gets too thick , add more water .
Remove it from the stove and let cool for 2-3
minutes
Serve it while is still warm.
This is a delicious and very nutritious meal for any
time of the day.
Try it you will like it.

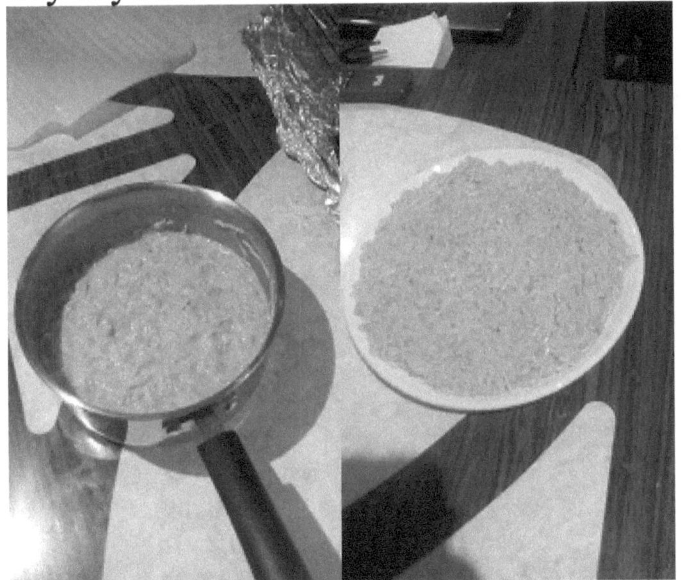

that's how it looks when you cook oats and
capellini with milk.

@@@@@@@@@@@@@@@@@@@@@@@@@
@@@@@@@

Recipe
Milk and rice

Ingredients

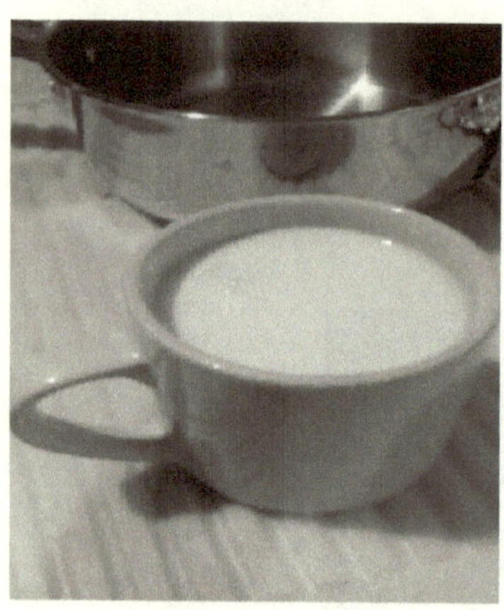
a cup of milk

2 cups of water
1 cup of 2% milk
1 cup of rice your choice.
3 table spoons of sugar or honey for sweetening
which is optional.

Pour the water and milk in a pot and place it on
the stove. Add the sugar and stir it to dissolve.

When the mixture starts to boil
 Rinse the rice and add the rice into the mixture
Lower the heat to medium and let it cook for 20-
25 minutes or until the rice is cooked.
Remove it from the stove, let it cool for a few
minutes and then put the cooked rice in small
containers and sprinkle some pulverized
cinnamon on it for aromatic taste, which is of
course optional. When the milk-rice cools down
you can put it in the fridge and serve it at any time
you want as a desert or a meal.

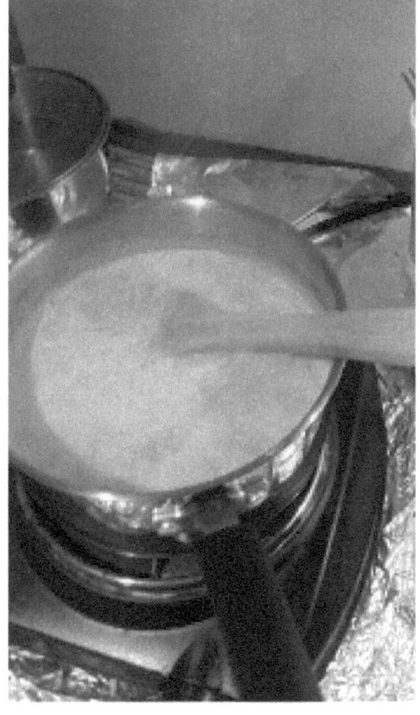

These are my personal recipes which are
nutritious and delicious as they contain all   the
necessary nutritional ingredients for good health
of your body.
I am sure you can find many other recipes in the

internet with milk or milk byproducts.

One cup of whole milk provides 276 milligrams of calcium 7.7 grams of protein and 4.5 grams of saturated fat for 149 calories. It also contains 322 milligrams of potassium , 205 milligrams of phosphorous , 24 milligrams of magnesium, and 0.9 milligrams of zinc 395 International Units (IU) of vitamin A. And, you'll find trace amounts of six B vitamins, including folate and b12, in milk.

In conclusion :

Milk is good for everybody unless they have allergy or milk intolerance in which case they should eat other calcium rich foods.

Milk for the babies.

 Make sure that babies get enough milk everyday for their normal development and avoid rickets. Rickets is a skeletal disorder that results from a lack of vitamin D, calcium, or phosphate. These nutrients are important for the development of strong, healthy bones. All these nutrients are found in the milk and prevents the condition rickets in children.

Milk has all the nutrients for the babies nutritional needs until they can have solid food.

Milk for kids :

Milk is essential for the normal growth of kids. They should drink milk everyday for good health of their bodies , bones and teeth. Milk prevents rickets in growing kids.

Milk for adults:

It is essential that adults drink milk too and other foods rich in calcium for their daily calcium requirements. A lack of calcium in adults can cause osteoporosis, bone fractures and other conditions mimicking dementia and Alzheimer's.

Milk for the sick; sick people should drink warm milk for fast recovery. Milk has the essential nutrients to help the body regain   strength .

Milk   for the aged:

it is absolutely necessary for people over 65 years of age to drink milk and eat foods rich in calcium to prevent osteoporosis and bone fractures. Severe symptoms of hypocalcaemia especially   to old people include:

Confusion and memory loss which can mimic

Alzheimer 's disease, depression, hallucinations, muscle cramps and numbness and tingling to the hands and feet.

There is a possibility that many old people that are diagnosed with dementia and Alzheimer's disease , suffer from hypocalcaemia or other nutritional deficiencies! It is about time that people over 65 to get milk in their daily diet and other nutritional foods.

@@@@@@@@@@@@@@@@@@@@@@@@
@@@

NUMBER TWO BEST FOOD IS EGGS.

Thank god to chickens and other birds that provide us with nutritious eggs which are   better than the golden eggs.

Eggs are very nutritious for everybody at any age.

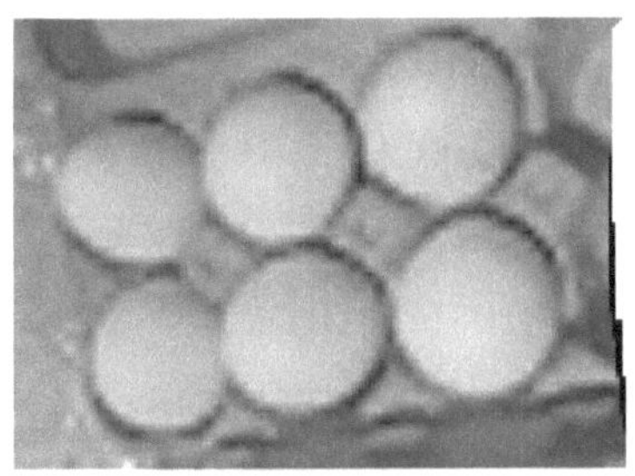

Eggs have all the nutrients to sustain life. Think of it this way, you have an egg and with the right conditions in 21 days a young healthy chick will come out from that egg, which means that the egg has everything necessary to create a new life, a new chick.

You can eat eggs at any time of the day as breakfast, lunch or dinner.

Eggs is a good source of high quality protein and other nutrients.

The nutritional value of eggs. I egg has 6 gr. Protein, total fat 5g, saturated fat 1.5g, cholesterol 185mg, sodium 70mg, vitamin D 1mcg,calcium 28mg, iron 1mg, potassium 69mg, riboflavin 0.2mg. Vitamin B12 0.4mg, biotin 10mcg, antithetic acid 1mg, iodine 27mcg, zinc 1mg, selenium 15mcg, molybdenum 8mcg,and choline 147mg . As we see eggs have all the nutrients necessary to sustain life and play an important role in muscle strength, brain function, eye health etc.

There are many recipes how to cook and eat eggs
and you should never eat raw eggs to prevent any
salmonella infection.
. The most common symptoms of salmonella
infections are diarrhea, fever, abdominal cramps,
and vomiting. This typically occurs between 12
hours and 36 hours after exposure and the
symptoms can last from two to seven days.
Occasionally the old, young, and others with a
weakened immune system are more likely to
develop severe disease resulting in dehydration
and a life threatening condition.

The best way to eat eggs is just boil them anyway
you like , hard boiled or soft eggs.
You can also fry the eggs but frying them increase
their calories from the oil that are fried in.
You can also make a delicious omelet with 2-3
eggs.
There so many ways to cook and eat eggs and if
you are interested in exotic recipes just look in the
internet.
If you just want to keep it fast and simple just boil
them from 3 to 7 minutes depending how you like
them. 3 minutes will be soft boiled eggs and 7
minutes will be hard boiled eggs. any way you eat
them are nutritious and that's the most important
thing to keep in mind.
People of all ages should eat eggs regularly for

good health.
Young kids should eat eggs everyday to keep them healthy.
of course people with egg allergy should not eat eggs and they should consult their doctor for advice.

For many years, the medical community was against eating eggs   due to their cholesterol content and   they were advising their patients to avoid eggs.   Because of that, many older patients stopped eating   the nutritional eggs and many of them developed nutritional deficiencies and even dementia.
Fortunately after many years of research the scientific community found that cholesterol content in the eggs is not as bad as they first thought and now they are advising patients to eat the nutritional eggs again but   in moderation.
Thank god for that, now older patients can eat eggs and other nutritional foods to avoid deficiencies.
Eggs are not only nutritional but are also reasonable priced and can be prepared easily and served as a breakfast, lunch and dinner. Eggs are also very good for people that want to loose weight or maintain their weight at a normal level.

@@@@@@@@@@@@@@@@@@@@@@@@@
@@@@@@@

Here are a few recipes how to eat eggs and benefit from their high nutritional value.

The easiest recipe is just boiled eggs which anybody can prepare in a few minutes.

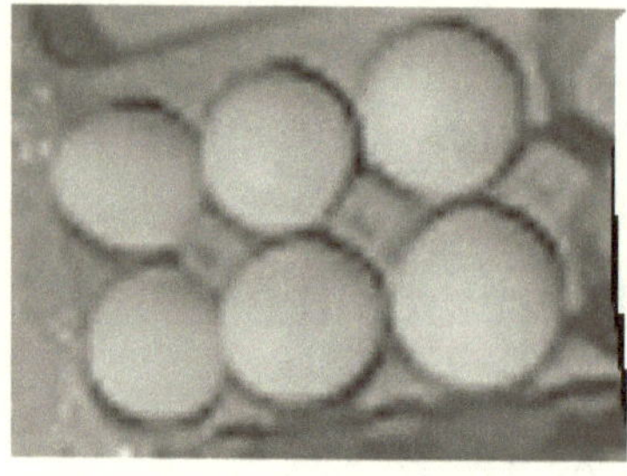

Two to three medium or large eggs

Put water in a small pot

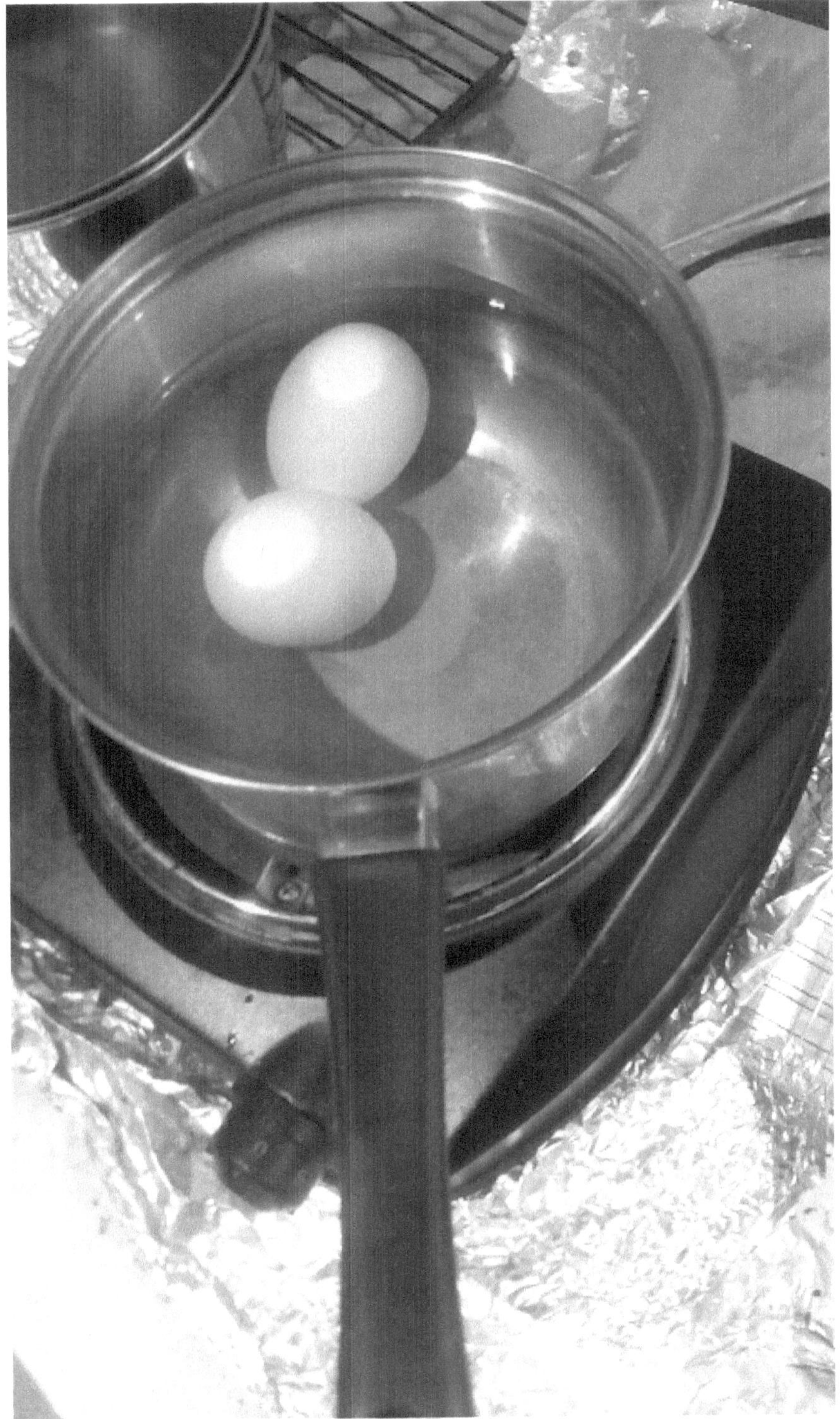

and place the eggs in the water
This is very important and if the eggs float on the
water it means that are spoiled and are not good to
eat them. Always keep your eggs in the fridge to
last longer.
Place the pot on the stove and turn it on
Let the water boil for 2 minutes for soft boiled
eggs
And 5minutes for hard boiled eggs
Remove the eggs from the boiling water and let
them cool down for a few minutes , or if you are
on a hurry just put them in cold water to cool.
You can eat the eggs with 1-2 whole wheat
toasts.

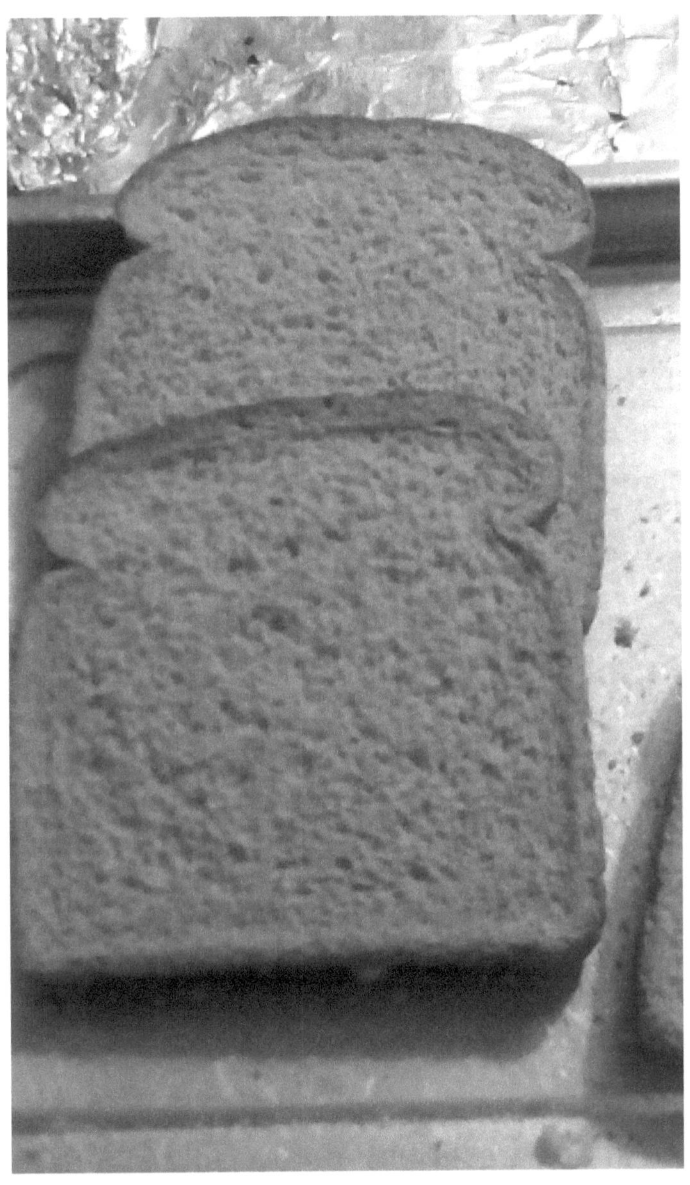

You can also eat eggs as a delicious omelet,
scrambled eggs, egg salads with hard boiled eggs,
or just put them in soups.

Anyway you decide to eat them are delicious and very nutritional.

 Eggs are supposed to be aphrodisiacs too. These aphrodisiacs not only increase your libido but also improve your sexual performance.
Eggs are rich in vitamins B1 & B2, which help with the production of sex hormones. In addition, they also have an effect on mood and metabolism since they contain iodine, manganese, and selenium.

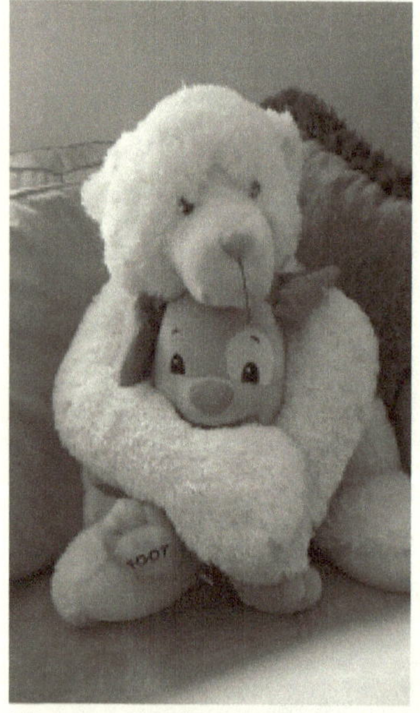

Eggs help men and women with their libido , so if you want your partner to be more sexually active feed them   some eggs on a regular basis, if there is no allergy present. Use eggs in your soups and other dishes.
Eggs enhance strength and endurance and many

athletes eat a lot of eggs before their performance.
I remember seeing some wrestlers ordering half
a dozen eggs each at the local restaurant for their
breakfast the day they had a wrestling match.

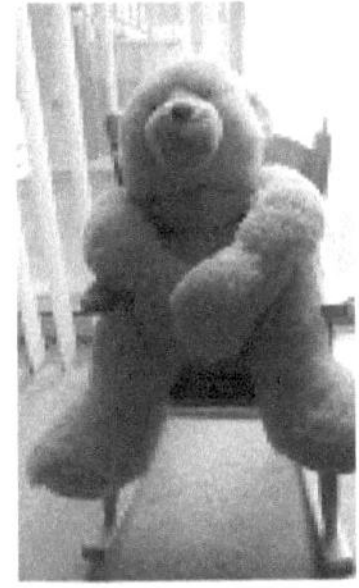

There are many recipes for eggs and you can look
them up in the internet if you are interested in fancy
and complicated recipes. Just remember that the
simpler the recipe is, the easier it is to follow.
If you are in a hurry and you want a nutritional
meal fast ,just boil half a dozen eggs and keep
them in the fridge to eat them any time you are
hungry.

@@@@@@@@@@@@@@@@@@@@@@@
@@@@

NUMBER THREE BEST FOOD IS WHOLE
WHEAT BREAD

As we have seen above , mother nature provided the best nutritional food for the live birth animals, their mothers' milk, it also provided all nutritional needs for the oviparous animals that come from the eggs and stored all the necessary nutrients in the seeds of plants, for the plant seedlings. Mother Nature takes care for the survival of the future generations by storing the necessary nutrients for the young until they are able to provide for themselves.

In the case of plants nature stores all the necessary nutrients for the young seedling until it grows its roots and can feed from the mother earth. In every single seed we find the germ, the future young embryo ready to break out when the conditions are favorable. In that seed we find the germ which is equivalent of the live embryo in the animal kingdom , the endosperm which is the food for the young embryo until it takes root, and a seed coat which is the protective cover for the embryo and its food and that protective coat is the wheat bran.

All plant seeds are a powerhouse full of all nutrients necessary to sustain life and the humans have chosen the plants seeds for their nutrition. Depending which part of the globe people live they choose and the prevalent seeds of that particular area for their food. In Asia the most prevalent seeds is rice so the people in those countries their favorite seed for food is rice. In most of the other countries their favorite seed for food is wheat which they make into many varieties of breads , cookies, cakes etc.   Can you imagine a world without the creation of the wheat products? No bread, no pasta, no cookies, no cakes, no cereal etc .

Wheat is a grass cultivated for its nutritional seed for many thousands of years. It is a cereal grain and a worldwide staple food. There are many species of wheat but the most widely grown is the common wheat used to feed the world.
Wheat is a very nutritional food and contains Vitamins such as thiamine (B1), riboflavin (B2), pantothenic acid, inosotol, P-aminobenzoic acid, folic acid and vitamin B6 .   With all the nutrients contained in the **wheat, it** makes **bread** an essential part of the world diet. Many people were saved from starvation during the great wars by eating just bread.

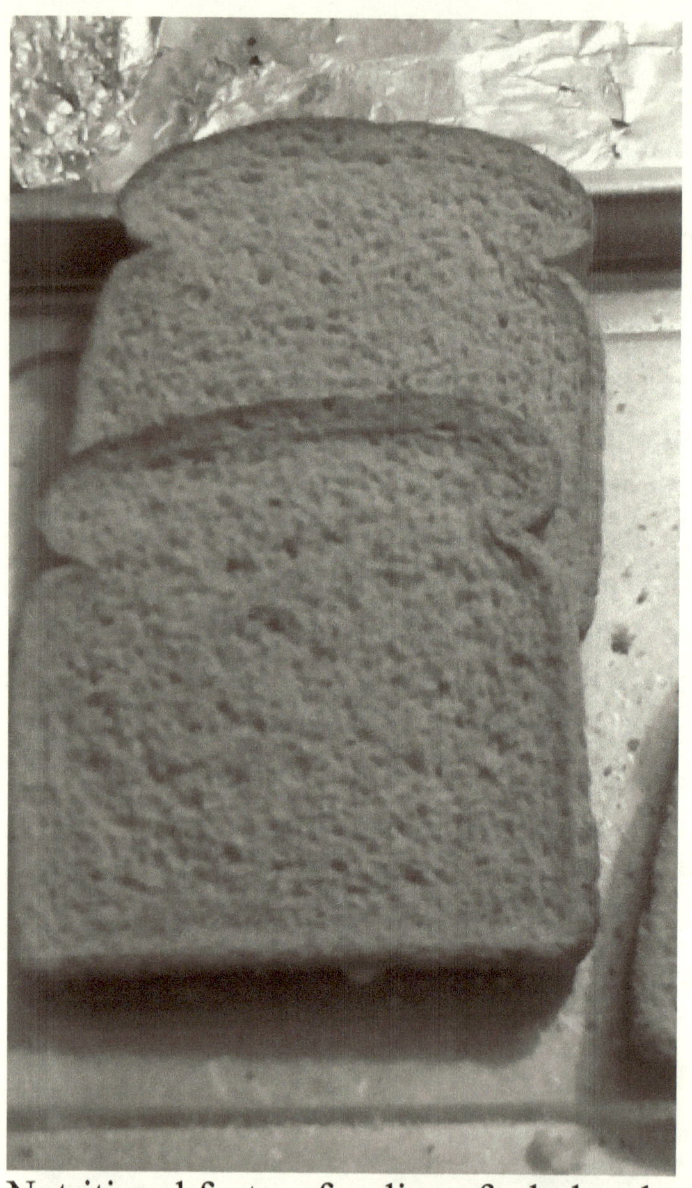

Nutritional facts of a slice of whole wheat bread :
 approximately 29 grams, total fat 1gr, saturated
fat 0.02 gr, sodium 110 mg, carbohydrates 11gr,
fiber 1gr, glucose 1gr, protein 3gr,
Calcium 20 mg, iron 0.3mg,

The structure of the wheat grain is 4-10mm long consisting of the germ , the endosperm and a seed coat which is the wheat bran. The endosperm is the potential white flour within the centre of the wheat grain, the nutritional needs of the embryo when it forms a new wheat plant. The Bran is nutritionally rich in protein and is used in the production of brown and whole meal flours.
The wheat germ is the embryo that would eventually develop into the new wheat plant. It is rich in vitamins, protein and oil and it is often used in health foods, such as fortified bread .. It's also a good source of magnesium, zinc, thiamin, folate, potassium, and phosphorus and high in vitamin E which has antioxidant properties.

The wheat germ and   wheat bran with their high nutritional value are sold in health food stores . When they used the whole wheat grain to make the whole wheat flour they make whole wheat bread which is very nutritious.
Flour is a powder made by grinding raw grains or roots and used to make many different foods.
 There are Different types of flour and its uses; there are several types of flour and from different sources but the only thing we are interested is the whole wheat flour which is used to make whole wheat bread which is an excellent   source of

nutrition for the human body. Whole wheat flour contains all three parts of the wheat seed , the germ, the endosperm and the bran which means that has all the nutrients of wheat.

As we mentioned previously, nature created the seeds which is a powerhouse for the nutritional needs of the future seedling and   humans take advantage of this fact to use seeds for their nutritional needs.   All kinds of seeds are used by humans to eat them or make flour for making bread or other uses. There are all sorts of flour made from different kinds of seeds in different parts of the globe. Even birds use seeds as their main food supply and some of them even store them for future consumption.

The most important thing to remember is that bread made from the whole wheat flour is very nutritious for the human body providing almost all essential nutrients, vitamins, minerals, protein and carbohydrates for good health.

When combining whole wheat bread with milk and eggs in our daily diets gives our bodies all the necessary nutrients for good health.

Make it a habit to eat whole wheat bread daily, unless you have an allergy or celiac disease in which case you can replace the whole wheat bread with other products which are equivalent to bread.

There are many other types of bread made from
edible grains like oats, corn, barley rye etc. and
you should always try to eat the bread that it is
made from the whole grain which includes the
germ, the endosperm and hull.
 There are breads made   with white flour where
the germ and the bran is removed making the
white breads but are not as nutritious as the whole
grain breads.

VEGETARIANS:

There are a lot of people that are vegetarians and
they never eat animal meat , fish or their products
and I am sure they have replaced the animal
proteins with plant proteins like legumes, nuts and
other products. There are many reasons why
people   become vegetarians and each and every
one have their own reason unless they are
unwillingly victims of other people choices and
influence, like being members of a cult ,their
parents or spouses?
Whatever the situation is, I think it is necessary to
include in their diet milk , eggs , whole wheat
bread and other foods which contain   all the

necessary nutrients to sustain life otherwise they
will develop nutritional deficiencies.
Of course it is their choice but the young and old
will be at risk of nutritional deficiency diseases.
If you have kids you have to give them nutritional
foods for proper development both physical and
mentally.

 NUMBER FOUR BEST FOOD IS MEAT,
CHICKEN, FISH,

All meats and fish are rich in high quality
complete protein and you should include them in
your diet. You do not have to buy the most
expensive piece of meat or fish but you should buy
the kind of meat you like to eat. Red **Meat** is
valued as a complete protein food containing all the
amino acids necessary for the human body. The fat

of **meat**, which varies widely with the species, quality, and cut, is a valuable source of energy. However too much fat consumption is not healthy and excess fat will be stored in the body as fat for future use and in the process might cause problems in the body's arteries arteriosclerosis and clogging of the arteries leading to health problems. It is better to choose lean meat and white meat like chicken and turkey meat and remove the skin and the excess visible fat.

Red or white meat for human consumption is essential for good health as it contains all amino acids needed by the human body to repair and regenerate the human cells.

You do not have to buy the most expensive cut of meat to benefit from the meat nutrition. Meat is a complete protein no matter which part of the animal part came from. If you are concerned about meat containing too much fat, you can eat chicken legs and breast and remove the skin which has fat and any other visible fat.

Turkey breast and legs are good source of meat by removing the skin and any visible fat.

You can also eat the animal organs, the liver, the spleen, the kidneys and even the brain. All the animal organs are packed with excellent nutrients which are good for your health. Liver and other organs have plenty of vitamins and minerals. You

can eat them well cooked alone , or in combination
with other foods such as soups.
 However if you do not like to eat animal organs
that's ok, you get all the essential nutrients for good
health from meat, milk, eggs and whole wheat
bread. Besides every one is different and has
different tastes. Some people enjoy eating animal
organs and others do not, and that is ok.

How to eat you meat? you have to cook it of course
and you should never eat it raw as it might contain
bacteria or other contaminants and make you sick.
You do not have to be a culinary chef to cook meat.
there are several ways to cook your meat and there
are plenty of recipes in the internet but the simplest
way is the easiest to cook.
The easiest way to cook your meat is just put it in
a cooking pot and add water and place on your
stove. You can add some peeled and cut carrots,
some garlic cloves , some onions and other
vegetables if you prefer and let it boil for half an
hour to an our until it is tender .
You can also roast it in the oven or barbeque it
.There are many ways to cook and eat meat with
plenty of recipes in the internet. I personally prefer
the easy simple way to just cook it in a pot with
water. By boiling the meat and some vegetables
you can get the broth and make soups which are
very nutritious and keep you warm especially in

the cold winder days.
Fish is very   good source of protein and other essential nutrients for good health. Some people like to eat a lot of fish and some of them avoid fish and that's a   personal choice . People that live in islands and do not have access to meat they supplement their diets with fishes which is a good replacement for meat. People from all over the world have learned to use whatever food source is readily available to them to feed their bodies for good health.

The purpose of this book is to emphasize that meat , fish, milk , eggs and whole wheat bread   are the best foods for good health and not to provide complicated recipes which you can easily find them in the internet
For vegetarians and other people that avoid to consume meat and fish, it is my hope that they get other nutritional foods that contain all essential proteins, vitamins and minerals that are needed by the body to function properly.

 Peoples' bodies react differently to different foods so it is very important to remember that if some foods do not agree with your body and make you feel uncomfortable, sick or have a reaction to a particular food you ate, just DO NOT EAT THAT FOOD AGAIN.

There is a saying that " a food can be poison for some people and medicine for others" , so it is up to each and every individual to find what food is good for them and what food is not good for them and avoid it.

OTHER FOODS THAT ARE GOOD FOR GOOD HEALTH

As we discuss above, milk, eggs, whole wheat bread and meat including fish are essential food for good health but you should also include in your diet other foods which although are not essential they do complement the above foods and they provide additional ingredients for optimum health. In your diet you should include edible nuts and almonds, legumes, beans, peas, lentils, fruits and vegetables to make delicious salads with olive oil and lemon.

Olive oil is the best edible oil , it is rich in energy, has vitamin E ,vitamin K, omega 3 , omega 6, and it is recommended by nutritionist as the healthiest oil for consumption. Olive oil is used in the Mediterranean diet which is considered one of the best diets for healthy living.

You should always eat food that agrees with your body. If you observe that one fruit, vegetable or other food gives you upset stomach or other unpleasant symptoms do not eat it. Eat only food that makes you feel good which means that agree with your body's need.

How to avoid food poisoning and other infections.

Food poisoning and other infections occur when the food you eat is spoiled or has some pathogenic bacteria like salmonella which is present in chicken and other foods. To avoid food infections you have to take the necessary precautions.
1)If the food you are about to eat looks bad, smell bad or has an unpleasant taste do not eat it! If you are doubt throw it out.
2) wash your hands with soap and water before you sit down to eat. Wash your hands after handling raw food including meat, fish eggs, vegetables and after touching the garbage bin or going to the washroom, or touch any pets .

**3)do not wash your meat or chicken in your kitchen sink as this can spread germs around your kitchen. Put your meat , chicken   in a pot of water and boil it. The boiling water will kill any bacteria present. if you intent to use that boiling water as your stock it is better to throw out the first water after the water boils for 5 to 10 minutes and replace it with new one.
4) keep your kitchen sink and working area clean.**

wash the worktops and sink.

5) use separate chopping boards , one for meat and another for the vegetables .

6)keep raw meats from the vegetables and store meats on the bottom shelf of the fridge.

7)keep your fridge temperature below 5C, This prevents harmful germs from growing and multiplying.

8) cook your food thoroughly and Make sure poultry, pork, burgers, sausages and kebabs are cooked until steaming hot, with no pink meat inside

9)Wash the dishcloths regularly, as Dirty, damp
cloths are the perfect place for germs to spread.

10) if you have any left over food refrigerate it as
soon as it cools down   and eat   it within 2 days or
use it for soups etc.
11)make sure to wash your vegetables in running
water and avoid using the same board you cut the
meat. make sure your cutting knife is clean from
any contamination with raw meat.

12)respect the " use-by" date, there is a reason
why they put that there. Harmful bacteria can
develop in the food after the expiry date. Do not
take any chance even if it looks good.

13) when you are dining out avoid salads or any
uncooked food. You never know if there are
bacteria in the salads or uncooked food, and you do
not know how long that food was left at room
temperature or if the handlers of that food had
clean hands.
When in doubt   leave it out!
14)if you are traveling, eat only well cooked food
and still hot food.
Heat kills the germs that cause diseases and that's
why you should eat well cooked food .
15) when traveling eat dry foods , bread, factory
sealed foods such as tuna . Avoid local restaurants

that look unsanitary.
Avoid tap water, go for bottled , canned or hot
drinks. Avoid local drinks with ice as there is a
chance for contamination .
16) always wash your hands before you eat
anything and   after Using the toilet , changing
diapers, coughing, sneezing or even
handshaking., handling, reptiles, birds or other
animals.
17) another source of infection and this might not
have to do with food poisoning ,is through personal
contact with someone that has an infection. To be
on the safe side , if you see someone with an
obvious signs of infection, cold, flu etc, avoid any
personal contact with them like hugging or shaking
hands. In my book : THE PROS AND CONS OF
HUGGING , I explained why people should avoid
hugging. If you shake hands with someone with
an infection make sure to wash your hands
thoroughly with soap and water.

If after taking all the above precautions you are
unlucky and get food poisoning with vomiting,
diarrhea , abdominal cramps and fever you better
see a doctor for proper diagnosis and treatments.
Usually food poisoning goes away in a few days
but you never know what bacteria   or virus
caused the food poisoning , so to be on the safe

side see your doctor . Some bacteria or viruses can cause life threatening diseases, so it is always advisable to see your trusted doctor or go the emergency department of the nearest hospital as soon as possible.

If you want to maintain or loose weight you should include these nutritious foods in your daily diet which are essential for optimum health. Always eat or drink in moderation. Excess eating or drinking can lead to problems in the long run . The ancient Greeks had this famous proverb: Pan metron Ariston :"Παν μέτρον άριστον ... "All things in **moderation**

In addition to good nutrition your body needs exercises to keep fit and it is a good idea to exercise daily. Exercising does not require expensive gym memberships or expensive equipment. Walking for 30 minutes daily is a good exercise. Swimming is an excellent exercise, or even working in your garden will give you plenty of exercising provided you take the necessary precautions to protect your low back from any injury.

 You can also do some spinal exercises like the ones I describe in my book: SCOLIOSIS: HOW TO PREVENT AND TREAT SCOLIOSIS WITH THE SPINAL ACTIVE FLEXION EXERCISES (S.A.F.E). Those exercises are good for anyone that has a spine and you can do them in the privacy of your home , even in your own bed.

CONCLUSION.

In conclusion, Food is essential for good health and choosing the right food it is a necessity. The aim of eating is not just to have a full stomach, but to eat the right foods that will give you all the necessary ingredients for optimum health. Milk , eggs, whole wheat bread , meat and fish dishes will provide all required nutrients for maintaining good health of your body. Complementing the above foods with fruits , vegetables , edible seeds and olive oil, your body should work like a well oiled machine.

 Proteins is the magic key for optimum health and the most important food for repairing and maintaining your body in good shape. Eat the right foods and you will be rewarded with good health

and even a long   healthy life   blessed with
happiness and the joy of healthy living.
Eating the right foods is no more expensive that
eating junk food, wasting money on drinking
alcohol, smoking or illegal drugs . On the contrary
nutritional foods like milk, eggs, whole wheat
bread, fish   and chicken meat is reasonably priced
and accessible to nay budget, rich or frugal.
I have emphasized the facts about the benefits
of eating good foods. Now it is up to you, if you
want to reap the health benefits of these foods .

The responsibility and the number one job of
every living creature is to keep their bodies in good
health by eating the right nutritional foods. It is my
hope that everybody knows that and make an
effort to provide their bodies with all the
necessary ingredients for optimum health by
choosing the right foods.

@@@@@@@@@@@@@@@@@@@@@@
@@@@@@@

Book description.
In this book I describe the most nutritional foods for good health for the young and the old.
If you want to eat nutritional foods for good health this book is for you.
If you suffer from constipation read this book to see what foods are good for that.
If you want your kids to eat nutritional foods and grow up healthy this book is a must read.
If you want your kids to do well in school give them the good foods I describe above.
If you suffer from insomnia try this easy recipe I describe in this book..
Healthy eating does not have to be expensive. Try these cheap highly nutritional foods for good health of your entire family.
Learn what are the most nutritional foods and how to eat them for good health.
Most athletes eat lots of these highly nutritious foods daily to keep them strong , healthy and above all competitive.
The responsibility and the number one job of every living creature is to keep their bodies in good health by eating the right nutritional foods. It is my hope that everybody knows that and make an effort to provide their bodies with all the necessary ingredients for optimum health by choosing the right foods.

To find out which foods have all the necessary
ingredients to keep your body in optimum health ,
 just click the BUY button   now and you will be
on your way to obtain the desirable results for
good health.